Plant Based Diet Recipes 2021

A Collection of Healthy Plant-Based Recipes for Losing Weight and Healthy Living for Beginners

Frank Smith

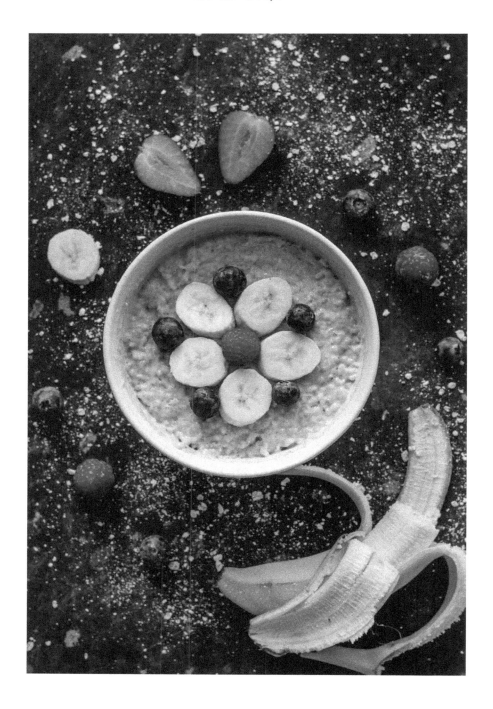

Table Of Contents

BREAKFASTS **8**

1   ONION & MUSHROOM TART WITH A NICE BROWN RICE CRUST 8

SOUPS, SALADS, AND SIDES **12**

2   CREAMY SQUASH SOUP 12

3   CUCUMBER EDAMAME SALAD 15

4   BEST BROCCOLI SALAD 18

ENTRÉES **20**

5   CRUNCHY ASPARAGUS SPEARS 20

6   CUCUMBER BITES WITH CHIVE AND SUNFLOWER SEEDS 23

SMOOTHIES AND BEVERAGES **26**

7   TANGY SPICED CRANBERRY DRINK 26

8   WARM POMEGRANATE PUNCH 29

9   RICH TRUFFLE HOT CHOCOLATE 31

10   VANILLA MILKSHAKE 33

11   RASPBERRY PROTEIN SHAKE 34

12   RASPBERRY ALMOND SMOOTHIE 35

13   APPLE RASPBERRY COBBLER 36

SNACKS AND DESSERTS 38

14   SIMPLE BANANA FRITTERS 38

15   COCONUT AND BLUEBERRIES ICE CREAM 41

16   PEACH CROCKPOT PUDDING 43

17   GREEN SOY BEANS HUMMUS 45

18   HIGH PROTEIN AVOCADO GUACAMOLE.....................47

19   HOMEMADE ENERGY NUT BARS 49

20   CHOCOLATE ENERGY SNACK BAR............................51

21   ZESTY ORANGE MUFFINS 53

22   CHOCOLATE TAHINI BALLS.....................................55

DINNER RECIPES 58

23   PIQUILLO SALSA VERDE STEAK 58

24   SWEET 'N SPICY TOFU 62

LUNCH RECIPES 64

25   GREEN PEA FRITTERS 64

26   BROCCOLI RABE 68

27   WHIPPED POTATOES..70

28   CHICKPEA AVOCADO SANDWICH 72

29   PIZZA BITES 74

30   AVOCADO, SPINACH AND KALE SOUP 76

31   CURRY SPINACH SOUP..78

32   HOT ROASTED PEPPERS CREAM 79

RECIPES FOR MAIN COURSES AND SINGLE DISHES......................... 82

33   SMOKED TEMPEH WITH BROCCOLI FRITTERS 82

34   CHEESY POTATO CASSEROLE 86

35   CURRY MUSHROOM PIE 88

NUTRIENT-PACKED PROTEIN SALADS 92

36   ARUGULA LENTIL SALAD 92

FLAVOUR BOOSTERS (FISH GLAZES, MEAT RUBS & FISH RUBS) ... 96

37   TUNISIAN MIXED SPICED RUB 96

38   ALL PURPOSE DILL SEED RUB 99

SAUCE RECIPES 102

39   VEGAN RANCH DRESSING (DIPPING SAUCE) 102

40   VEGAN SMOKEY MAPLE BBQ SAUCE 104

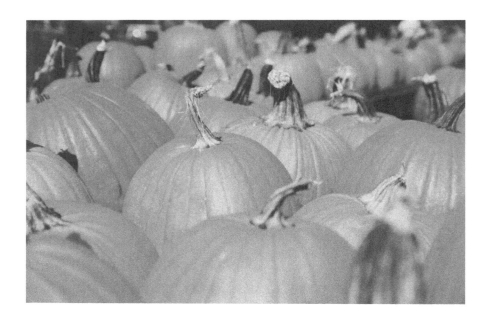

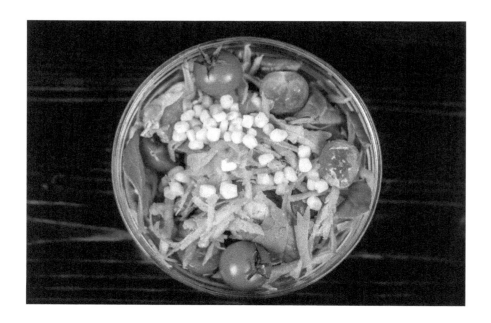

Breakfasts

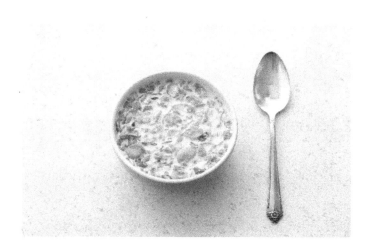

1 Onion & Mushroom Tart with a Nice Brown Rice Crust

Preparation 10 minutesCooking 55 minutes Serving: 1

Ingredients:

1 ½ pounds, mushrooms, button, portabella,1 cup, short-grain brown rice

2 ¼ cups, water

½ teaspoon, ground black pepper 2 teaspoons, herbal spice blend 1 sweet large onion 7 ounces, extra-firm tofu

1 cup, plain non-dairy milk 2 teaspoons, onion powder

2 teaspoons, low-sodium soy1 teaspoon, molasses

¼ teaspoon, ground turmeric ¼ cup, white wine

¼ cup, tapiocaDirections:

Cook the brown rice and put it aside for later use.

Slice the onions into thin strips and sauté them in water until they aresoft. Then, add the molasses, and cook them for a few minutes.

Next, sauté the mushrooms in water with the herbal spice

blend. Once the mushrooms are cooked and they are soft, add the white wine or sherry. Cook everything for a few more minutes.

In a blender, combine milk, tofu, arrowroot, turmeric, and onionpowder till you have a smooth mixture

On a pie plate, create a layer of rice, spreading evenly to form a crust. The rice should be warm and not cold. It will be easy to work with warm rice. You can also use a pastry roller to get an even crust. With your fingers, gently press the sides.

Take half of the tofu mixture and the mushrooms and spoon them over the tart dish. Smooth the level with your spoon.

Now, top the layer with onions followed by the tofu mixture. You can smooth the surface again with your spoon.

Sprinkle some black pepper on top.

Bake the pie at 350o F for about 45 minutes. Toward the end, you can cover it loosely with tin foil. This will help the crust to remain moist.

Allow the pie crust to cool down, so that you can slice it.

If you are in love with vegetarian dishes, there is no way that you will not love thispie.

Nutrition: Calories: 245.3, Fats 16.4 g, Proteins 6.8 g, Carbohydrates 18.3 g

Soups, Salads, and Sides

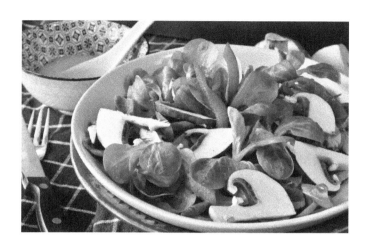

2 Creamy Squash Soup

Preparation time: 35 minutes Cooking time: 22 minutes

Servings: 8

Ingredients:

3 cups butternut squash, chopped

1 ½ cups unsweetened coconut milk1 tbsp coconut oil

1 tsp dried onion flakes1 tbsp curry powder

4 cups water

1 garlic clove

1 tsp kosher saltDirections:

Add squash, coconut oil, onion flakes, curry powder, water, garlic, and salt into a large saucepan. Bring to boil over high heat.

Turn heat to medium and simmer for 20 minutes.

Puree the soup using a blender until smooth. Return soup to the saucepan and stir in coconut milk and cook for 2 minutes.

Stir well and serve hot.

Nutrition: calories 146; fat 12.6 g; carbohydrates 9.4 g;

sugar 2.8 g;

protein 1.7 g; cholesterol 0 mg

3 Cucumber Edamame Salad

Preparation time: 5 minutes Cooking time: 8 minutes

Servings: 2

Ingredients:

3 tbsp. Avocado oil

1 cup cucumber, sliced into thin rounds

½ cup fresh sugar snap peas, sliced or whole

½ cup fresh edamame

¼ cup radish, sliced

1 large avocado, peeled, pitted, sliced 1 nori sheet, crumbled

2 tsp. Roasted sesame seeds1 tsp. Salt

Directions:

Bring a medium-sized pot filled halfway with water to a boil overmedium-high heat.

Add the sugar snaps and cook them for about 2 minutes.

Take the pot off the heat, drain the excess water, transfer the sugar snaps to a medium-sized bowl and set aside for now.

Fill the pot with water again, add the teaspoon of salt and bring to aboil over medium-high heat.

Add the edamame to the pot and let them cook for about 6 minutes.

Take the pot off the heat, drain the excess water, transfer

the soybeans to the bowl with sugar snaps and let them cool down for about 5 minutes.

Combine all ingredients, except the nori crumbs and roasted sesameseeds, in a medium-sized bowl.

Carefully stir, using a spoon, until all ingredients are evenly coated in oil. Top the salad with the nori crumbs and roasted sesame seeds.

Transfer the bowl to the fridge and allow the salad to cool for at least30 minutes.

Serve chilled and enjoy!

Nutrition: Calories 409 Carbohydrates 7.1 g Fats 38.25 g Protein 7.6g

4 Best Broccoli Salad

Preparation time: 15 minutes Chilling time: 1 hour

Servings: 8

Ingredients:

8 cups diced broccoli

¼ cup sunflower seeds

3 tablespoons apple cider vinegar

½ cup dried cranberries1/3 cup cubed onion

1 cup mayonnaise

½ cup bacon bits

2 tablespoons sugar

½ teaspoon salt and ground black pepperDirections:

In a bowl, mix vinegar, salt, pepper, mayonnaise, and sugar. Mix it

well. In another bowl, mix all the remaining ingredients and pour the prepared mayonnaise dressing and mix it well. Before serving to refrigerate it for at least an hour.

Nutrition: Carbohydrates 17g, protein 6g, fats 26g, calories 317

Entrées

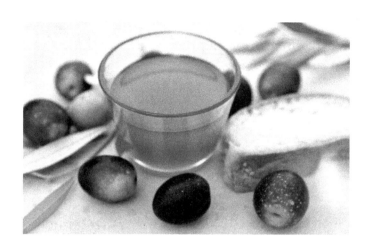

5 Crunchy Asparagus Spears

Preparation time: 25 minutes Cooking time: 25 minutes

Servings: 4

Ingredients:

1 bunch asparagus spears (about 12 spears)

¼ cup nutritional yeast

2 tablespoons hemp seeds1 teaspoon garlic powder

¼ teaspoon paprika (or more if you like paprika)

⅛ teaspoon ground pepper

¼ cup whole-wheat breadcrumbsJuice of ½ lemon

Directions:

Preheat the oven to 350 degrees, Fahrenheit.   Lin

Wash the asparagus, snapping off the white part at the bottom.Save it for making vegetable stock.

Mix together the nutritional yeast, hemp seed, garlic powder, paprika,pepper and breadcrumbs.

Place asparagus spears on the baking sheets giving them a little room in between and sprinkle with the mixture in the bowl.

Bake for up to 25 minutes, until crispy.

Serve with lemon juice if desired.

6 Cucumber Bites with Chive and Sunflower Seeds

Preparation time: 5 minutes Cooking time: 5 minutes

Servings: 2

Ingredients:

1 cup raw sunflower seed ½ teaspoon salt

½ cup chopped fresh chives1 clove garlic, chopped

2 tablespoons red onion, minced

2 tablespoons lemon juice

½ cup water (might need more or less)4 large cucumbers

Directions:

Place the sunflower seeds and salt in the food processor

and process to a fine powder. It will take only about 10 seconds.

Add the chives, garlic, onion, lemon juice and water and process until creamy, scraping down the sides frequently. The mixture shouldbe very creamy; if not, add a little more water.

Cut the cucumbers into 1½-inch coin-like pieces.

Spread a spoonful of the sunflower mixture on top and set on a platter. Sprinkle more chopped chives on top and refrigerate until

ready to serve.

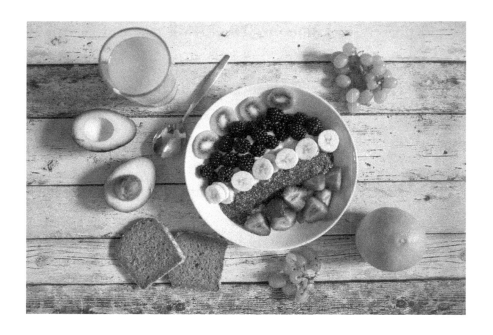

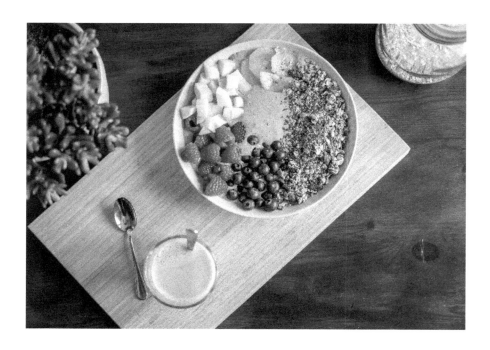

Smoothies and Beverages

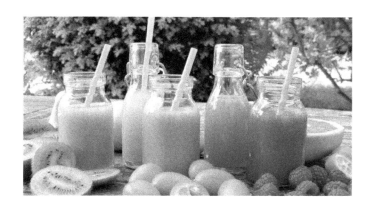

7 Tangy Spiced Cranberry Drink

Preparation time: 3 hours and 10 minutes Cooking time: 3

hours

Servings: 14

Ingredients:

1 1/2 cups of coconut sugar12 whole cloves

2 fluid ounce of lemon juice

6 fluid ounce of orange juice

32 fluid ounce of cranberry juice8 cups of hot water

1/2 cup of Red Hot candies

Directions:

Pour the water into a 6-quarts slow cooker along with the cranberryjuice, orange juice, and the lemon juice.

Stir the sugar properly.

Wrap the whole cloves in a cheese cloth, tie its corners with strings,and immerse it in the liquid present inside the slow cooker.

Add the red hot candies to the slow cooker and cover it

with the lid.

Then plug in the slow cooker and let it cook on the low

heat settingfor 3 hours or until it is heated thoroughly.

When done, discard the cheesecloth bag and serve.

Nutrition: Calories:89 Cal, Carbohydrates:27g,

Protein:0g, Fats:0g,Fiber:1g.

8 Warm Pomegranate Punch

Preparation: 3 hours and 15 minutes Cooking: 3 hours

Servings: 10

Ingredients:

3 cinnamon sticks, each about 3 inches long 12 whole cloves

1/2 cup of coconut sugar 1/3 cup of lemon juice

32 fluid ounce of pomegranate juice

32 fluid ounce of apple juice, unsweetened 16 fluid ounce of brewed tea

Directions:

Using a 4-quart slow cooker, pour the lemon juice,

pomegranate, juice apple juice, tea, and then sugar.

Wrap the whole cloves and cinnamon stick in a cheese cloth, tie its corners with a string, and immerse it in the liquid present in the slow cooker.

Then cover it with the lid, plug in the slow cooker and let it cook atthe low heat setting for 3 hours or until it is heated thoroughly.

When done, discard the cheesecloth bag and serve it hot or cold.

Nutrition: Calories:253 Cal, Carbohydrates:58g, Protein:7g, Fats:2g,Fiber:3g.

9 Rich Truffle Hot Chocolate

Preparation time: 2 hours and 10 minutes Cooking time: 2 hours

Servings: 4

Ingredients:

1/3 cup of cocoa powder, unsweetened 1/3 cup of coconut sugar 1/8 teaspoon of salt

1/8 teaspoon of ground cinnamon

1 teaspoon of vanilla extract, unsweetened 32 fluid ounce of coconut milk

Directions:

Using a 2 quarts slow cooker, add all the ingredients and

stirproperly.

Cover it with the lid, then plug in the slow cooker and cook it for 2hours on the high heat setting or until it is heated thoroughly.

When done, serve right away.

Nutrition: Calories:67 Cal, Carbohydrates:13g, Protein:2g, Fats:2g,Fiber:2.3g.

10 Vanilla Milkshake

Preparation: 5 min.Cooking: 5 min.Servings: 4

Ingredients:

2 c. ice cubes 2 t. vanilla extract

6 tbsp. powdered erythritol1 c. cream of dairy-free

½ c. coconut milkDirections:

In a high-speed blender, add all the ingredients and blend.

Add ice cubes and blend until smooth.

Serve immediately and enjoy!

Nutrition: Calories: 125 | Carbohydrates: 6.8 g |

Proteins: 1.2 g |Fats: 11.5 g

11 Raspberry Protein Shake

Preparation: 5 min. Cooking: 5 min.Serving: 1 Ingredients:

¼ avocado 1 c. raspberries, frozen1 scoop protein powder

½ c. almond milk

Ice cubes Directions:

In a high-speed blender add all the ingredients and blend

until lumpsof fruit disappear.

Add two to four ice cubes and blend to your desired

consistency.Serve immediately and enjoy!

Nutrition: Calories: 756 | Carbohydrates: 80.1 g |

Proteins: 27.6 g |

Fats: 40.7 g

12 Raspberry Almond Smoothie

Preparation: 5 min.Cooking: 5 min.Serving: 1

Ingredients:

10 Almonds, finely chopped3 tbsp. almond butter

1 c. almond milk 1 c. Raspberries, frozenDirections:

In a high-speed blender, add all the ingredients and

blend until

smooth.

Serve immediately and enjoy!

Nutrition: Calories: 449 | Carbohydrates: 26 g | Proteins:

14 g | Fats:35 g

13   Apple Raspberry Cobbler

Preparation Time: 50 minutesServings: 4

A safer type of fruit cobbler where a cut in sugar enhances the fruit.Ingredients

3 apples, peeled, cored, and chopped 2 tbsp pure date sugar cup fresh raspberries

1 tbsp unsalted plant butter

½ cup whole-wheat flour 1 cup toasted rolled oats 2 tbsp pure date sugar 1 tsp cinnamon powderDirections

Preheat the oven to 350 F and grease a baking dish with some plantbutter.

Add the apples, date sugar, and 3 tbsp of water to a medium pot. Cook over low heat until the date sugar melts and then, mix in the raspberries. Cook until the fruits soften, 10 minutes.

Pour and spread the fruit mixture into the baking dish and set aside. In a blender, add the plant butter, flour, oats, date sugar, and cinnamon powder. Pulse a few times until crumbly.

Spoon and spread the mixture on the fruit mix until evenly layered. Bake in the oven for 25 to 30 minutes or until golden brown on top. Remove the dessert, allow cooling for 2 minutes, and serve.

Nutritional info per serving

Calories 539 | Fats 12g| Carbs 105.7g | Protein 8.2g

Snacks and Desserts

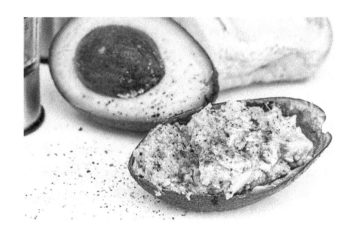

14 Simple Banana Fritters

Preparation time: 15 minsCooking time: 20 mins Servings:

8

Ingredients4 Bananas

3 Tbsps. Maple Syrup

¼ Tsp. Cinnamon Powder

¼ Tsp. Nutmeg

1 Cup Coconut FlourDirections

Preheat oven to 350° F.

Mash the bananas in a large mixing bowl along with maple syrup, cinnamon, nutmeg powder and coconut flour.

Mix all the ingredients well.

Take 2 tbsps. mixture and make small 1-inch-thick fritters from thismixture.

Place fritters in greased baking tray.

Bake fritters in preheated oven for about 10-15 minutes until goldenfrom both sides.

Once done, take them out of the oven.Serve with coconut

cream.

Enjoy!

Nutrition: Protein: 3% 3 kcal Fat: 28% 30 kcal

Carbohydrates: 69%

75 kcal

15 Coconut And Blueberries Ice Cream

Preparation time: 5 minsCooking time: 0 mins Servings: 4

Ingredients

1/4 Cup Coconut Cream1 Tbsp. Maple Syrup

¼ Cup Coconut Flour

1 Cup Blueberries

¼ Cup Blueberries For ToppingDirections

Put ingredients into food processor and mix well on high speed.

Pour mixture in silicon molds and freeze in freezer for about 2-4hours.

Once balls are set remove from freezer.Top with berries.

Serve cold and enjoy!

Nutrition: Protein: 3% 4 kcal Fat: 40% 60 kcal

Carbohydrates: 57%

86 kcal

16 Peach Crockpot Pudding

Preparation time: 15 minsCooking time: 4 hours Servings:

6

Ingredients

2 Cups Sliced Peaches1/4 Cup Maple Syrup

1/2 Tsp. Cinnamon Powder

2 Cups Coconut MilkFor Serving

½ Cup Coconut Cream1 Oz. Coconut Flakes Directions

Lightly grease the crockpot and place peaches in the

bottom.Add maple syrup, cinnamon powder and milk.

Cover and cook on high for 4 hours.

Once cooked remove from crockpot. For serving pour

coconut cream.

Top with coconut flakes.Serve and enjoy!

Nutrition: Protein: 3% 11 kcal Fat: 61% 230 kcal

Carbohydrates: 36%

133 kcal

17 Green Soy Beans Hummus

Preparation time: 15 minutes Cooking time: 0 minutes

Servings: 6

Ingredients

1 1/2 cups frozen green soybeans4 cups of water

coarse salt to taste

1/4 cup sesame paste 1/2 tsp grated lemon peel 3 Tbsp

fresh lemon juice 2 cloves of garlic crushed1/2 tsp ground

cumin

1/4 tsp ground coriander

4 Tbsp extra virgin olive oil

1 Tbsp fresh parsley leaves chopped

Serving options: sliced cucumber, celery, olivesDirections:

1. In a saucepan, bring to boil 4 cups of water with 2 to 3 pinch ofcoarse salt.

2. Add in frozen soybeans, and cook for 5 minutes or until tender.

3. Rinse and drain soybeans into a colander.

4. Add soybeans and all remaining ingredients into a food processor.

5. Pulse until smooth and creamy.

6. Taste and adjust salt to taste.

7. Serve with sliced cucumber, celery, olives, bread...etc.

18 High Protein Avocado Guacamole

Preparation time: 15 minutes Cooking time: 0 minutes

Servings: 4

Ingredients

1/2 cup of onion, finely chopped

1 chili pepper (peeled and finely chopped) 1 cup tomato,

finely chopped Cilantro leaves, fresh2 avocados

2 Tbsp linseed oil 1/2 cup ground walnuts 1/2 lemon (or

lime) Salt

Directions:

Chop the onion, chili pepper, cilantro, and tomato;

place in a largebowl.

Slice avocado, open vertically, and remove the pit. Using the spoon take out the avocado flesh.

Mash the avocados with a fork and add into the bowl with onionmixture.

Add all remaining ingredients and stir well until ingredients combinewell.

Taste and adjust salt and lemon/lime juice.

Keep refrigerated into covered glass bowl up to 5 days.

19 Homemade Energy Nut Bars

Preparation time: 15 minutes Cooking time: 0 minutes

Servings: 4

Ingredients

1/2 cup peanuts1 cup almonds

1/2 cup hazelnut, chopped

1 cup shredded coconut1 cup almond butter

2 tsp sesame seeds toasted

1/2 cup coconut oil, freshly melted2 Tbsp organic honey

1/4 tsp cinnamon

Directions

Add all nuts into a food processor and pulse for 1-2

minutes.

Add in shredded coconut, almond butter, sesame seeds, melted coconut oil, cinnamon, and honey; process only for one minute.

Cover a square plate/tray with parchment paper and apply the nutmixture.

Spread mixture vigorously with a spatula. Place in the freezer for 4 hours or overnight.

Remove from the freezer and cut into rectangular bars.

Ready! Enjoy!

20 Chocolate Energy Snack Bar

Preparation Time: 5 MinutesCooking Time: 0 Minutes

Servings: 4Ingredients:

Flax Seeds (1 T.)

Chia Seeds (1 T.) Agave Nectar (2 T.)Almonds (1 C.)

Dried Cranberries (1 C.)Dates (1 C.)

Directions:

When you need a snack that is easy to grab when you are on the go, this is the perfect recipe. You are going to start out by pulsing the almonds and dates in a food processor. Once they are chopped fine, add in the seeds, agave, and cranberries. At this point, pulse until everything is combined.

Next, you will want to add the batter into a lined pan and press everything down into the bottom.

Finally, pop the dish into the fridge for two hours, cut into squares, and your bars are ready!

Nutrition: Calories: 400 Proteins: 10g Carbs: 55g Fats: 20g

21 Zesty Orange Muffins

Preparation Time: 40 Minutes Cooking Time: 20 Minutes

Servings: 11

Ingredients:

Chopped Hazelnuts (3 T.)Orange Juice (1 C.)

Olive Oil (.50 C.)

Baking Powder (2 t.) Brown Sugar (.75 C.)Flour (2 C.)

Baking Soda (1 Pinch)Salt (to Taste)

Orange Zest (2 T.)

Directions:

Muffins are the perfect snack to grab and go when you

need to leave the house quickly. Start off by prepping the

oven to 350.

As this warms up, take out your mixing bowl and combine the hazelnuts, salt, baking soda, baking powder, sugar, and flour. Once these are mixed together well, add in the olive oil and orange juice.

With your mixture made, evenly pour into lined muffin tins and then pop it into the oven for 20 minutes.

By the end, the muffins should be cooked through and golden at the top. If they look done, remove from the oven, and your snack isready to go.

Nutrition: Calories: 220 Proteins: 3g Carbs: 30g Fats: 10g

22 Chocolate Tahini Balls

Preparation Time: 10 Minutes Cooking Time: 0 Minutes

Servings: 8

Ingredients:

Sesame Seeds (2 T.)Tahini (2 T.)

Cacao Nibs (2 T.)

Unsweetened Cocoa Powder (2 T.) Old-fashioned Rolled

Oats (.25 C.)Medjool Dates (4)

Rock Salt (1 Pinch)Directions:

For this quick snack, start off by placing all of the

ingredients aboveinto a blender and blend until you get a

dough-like texture.

Next, take the dough and mold it into 8 balls.

Place the balls in the fridge, allow to firm up for 20 minutes, and thenthey will be set.

Nutrition: Calories: 70 Proteins: 2g Carbs: 9g Fats: 4g

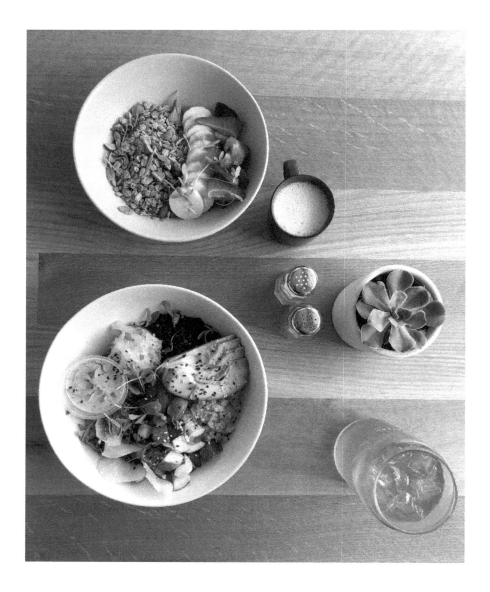

Dinner Recipes

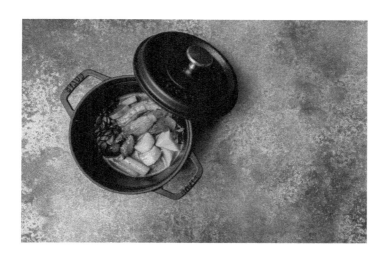

23 Piquillo Salsa Verde Steak

Preparation Time: 30 min.Cooking Time: 25 min.

Yields: 8 Servings

Ingredients:

4 – ½ inch thick slices of ciabatta18 oz. firm tofu, drained

5 tbsp. olive oil, extra virgin

Pinch of cayenne

½ t. cumin, ground

1 ½ tbsp. sherry vinegar1 shallot, diced

8 piquillo peppers (can be from a jar) – drained and cut to ½ inchstrips

3 tbsp. of the following:

parsley, finely chopsed capers, drained and chopped

Directions:

Place the tofu on a plate to drain the excess liquid, and then sliceinto 8 rectangle pieces.

You can either prepare your grill or use a grill pan. If using a grill pan,preheat the grill pan.

Mix 3 tablespoons of olive oil, cayenne, cumin, vinegar, shallot, parsley, capers, and piquillo peppers in a medium bowl to make our salsa verde. Season to preference with salt and pepper.

Using a paper towel, dry the tofu slices.

Brush olive oil on each side, seasoning with salt and pepper lightly.

Place the bread on the grill and toast for about 2 minutes usingmedium-high heat.

Next, grill the tofu, cooking each side for about 3 minutes or until thetofu is heated through.

Place the toasted bread on the plate then the tofu on top of thebread.

Gently spoon out the salsa verde over the tofu and serve.

Nutrition: Calories: 427 | Carbohydrates: 67.5 g |

Proteins: 14.2 g | Fats: 14.6 g

24 Sweet 'n spicy tofu

Preparation time 45 minutes Cooking time: 10 minutes

Servings: 8

Ingredients:

14 ounces extra firm tofu; press the excess liquid and chop intocubes.

3 tablespoons olive oil

2 2-3 cloves garlic, minced

4 tablespoons sriracha sauce or any other hot sauce 2 tablespoons soy sauce

1/4 cup sweet chili sauce

5-6 cups mixed vegetables of your choice (like carrots,

cauliflower,broccoli, potato, etc.)

Salt to taste (optional)Direction:

Place a nonstick pan over medium-high heat. Add 1 tablespoon oil.

When oil is hot, add garlic and mixed vegetables and stir-fry until crisp and tender. Remove and keep aside.

Place the pan back on heat. Add 2 tablespoons oil. When oil is hot, add tofu and sauté until golden brown. Add the sautéed vegetables. Mix well and remove from heat.

Make a mixture of sauces by mixing together all the sauces in asmall bowl.

Serve the stir fried vegetables and tofu with sauce.

Lunch Recipes

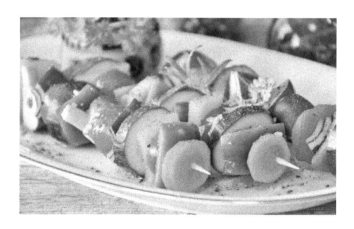

25 Green Pea Fritters

Preparation Time: 10 minutes Cooking Time: 25 minutes

Serving: 4

Ingredients:

For the Fritters:

1 ½ cups (140 grams) chickpea flour 2 cups (250 grams)

frozen peas

1 large white onion, peeled, diced

1 tablespoon minced garlic1/8 teaspoon salt

1 teaspoon baking soda

2 tablespoons mixed dried Italian herbs1 tablespoon olive oil

Water as needed

For the Yoghurt Sauce:

1/2 teaspoon dried rosemary 1/2 teaspoon dried parsley

1/2 teaspoon dried mint

1 lemon, juiced 1 cup soy yogurtDirections:

Switch on the oven, set it to 350° F and let it preheat.

Take a medium saucepan, place it over medium heat, add peas, cover them with water, bring it to a boil, cook for 2 to 3 minutes until tender, and when done, drain the peas and set aside until required.

Take a frying pan, place it over medium heat, add oil and when hot, add onion and garlic; cook for 5 minutes until softened.

Transfer onion-garlic mixture to a food processor, add peas and pulse for 1 minute until the thick paste comes together.

Tip the mixture in a bowl, add salt, baking soda, Italian herbs, and chickpea flour, stir until incorporated and shape the mixture into ten patties.

Brush the patties with oil, arrange them onto a baking sheet and bake for 15 to 18 minutes until golden brown and thoroughly cooked,turning halfway.

Meanwhile, prepare the yogurt sauce: take a medium bowl, add all the ingredients for it and whisk until combined.

Serve fritters with prepared yogurt sauce.

Nutrition: 94 Cal; 2 g Fat; 0 g Saturated Fat; 14 g Carbs; 3 g Fiber; 4 g Protein; 2 g Sugar

26 Broccoli Rabe

Preparation Time: 15 minutes Cooking Time: 15 minutes

Servings: 8

Ingredients:

2 oranges, sliced in half1 lb. broccoli rabe

2 tablespoons sesame oil, toasted

Salt and pepper to taste

1 tablespoon sesame seeds, toastedDirection

Pour the oil into a pan over medium heat.

Add the oranges and cook until caramelized. Transfer to a plate.

Put the broccoli in the pan and cook for 8 minutes.

Squeeze the oranges to release juice in a bowl.

Stir in the oil, salt and pepper.

Coat the broccoli rabe with the mixture. Sprinkle seeds on top.

Nutrition: Calories: 59 Total fat: 4.4g   Saturated fat: 0.6g Sodium:

164mg   Potassium: 160mg Carbohydrates: 4.1g Fiber: 1.6g Sugar:2g Protein: 2.2g

27 **Whipped Potatoes**

Preparation Time: 20 minutes Cooking Time: 35 minutes

Servings: 10

Ingredients:

4 cups water

3 lb. potatoes, sliced into cubes3 cloves garlic, crushed

6 tablespoons vegan butter2 bay leaves

10 sage leaves

½ cup Vegan yogurt

¼ cup low-fat milkSalt to taste Direction

Boil the potatoes in water for 30 minutes or until tender.

Drain.

In a pan over medium heat, cook the garlic in butter for 1 minute.

Add the sage and cook for 5 more minutes. Discard the garlic.

Use a fork to mash the potatoes.

Whip using an electric mixer while gradually adding the butter,yogurt, and milk.

Season with salt.

Nutrition: Calories: 169 Total fat: 7.6g Saturated fat: 4.7g

Cholesterol: 21mg Sodium: 251mg Potassium: 519mg

Carbohydrates: 22.1g Fiber: 1.5g Sugar: 2g Protein: 4.2g

28 **Chickpea Avocado Sandwich**

You can make the chickpea and avocado filling ahead of time and store it in the cold-storage box for or in the icebox. While avocado does brown easily, the lime juice helps preserve the integrity of it.

Preparation time: 10 minutes Cooking Time: 5 minutes

Servings: 2

Ingredients: Chickpeas – 1 canAvocado – 1

Dill, dried – .25 teaspoon Onion powder – .25 teaspoon

Sea salt – .5 teaspoon Celery, chopped – .25 cup

Green onion, chopped – .25 cup Lime juice – 3 tablespoons Garlic powder – .5 teaspoon Dark pepper, ground – dash Tomato, sliced – 1

Lettuce – 4 leavesBread – 4 slices Directions:

Drain the canned chickpeas and rinse them under cool water. Place them in a bowl along with the herbs, spices, sea salt, avocado, and lime juice. Using a potato masher or fork, mash the avocado and chickpeas together until you have a thick filling. Try not to mash the chickpeas all the way, as they create texture.Stir the celery and green onion into the filling and prepare yoursandwiches.

Layout two slices of bread, top them with the chickpea filling, some lettuce, and sliced tomato. Top them off with the two remainingslices, slice the sandwiches in half, and serve. Nutrition: Calories 471

29 Pizza Bites

Preparation Time: 1 Hour Cooking Time: 30 Minutes

Servings: 4

Ingredients:

Olive Oil (1 t.)

Dried Oregano (1 t.) Lemon Juice (1 t.) Dried Basil (1 t.)

Tomato Sauce (1 C.)Cauliflower (1 Head)Salt (to Taste)

Nutritional Yeast (to Taste) Garlic Cloves (2, Minced)

Directions:

Begin by prepping the oven to 300 and line a pan with

parchment paper. When this is set, take a mixing bowl and

combine the olive oil, oregano, basil, salt, tomato sauce,

and the basil together. In a second bowl, you will want to

place your nutritional yeast.

When you are ready, gently dip the cauliflower pieces into the tomatosauce and then roll in the nutritional yeast. You will want to place these on the baking sheet and continue until all of the cauliflower is covered.

Once the cauliflower is set, place it into the oven for about an hour oruntil the edges are crispy. Once they are cooked to your liking, remove from the oven and enjoy with some extra sauce for dipping!

Nutrition: Calories: 110 Proteins: 5g Carbs: 17g Fats: 3g

30 Avocado, Spinach and Kale Soup

Preparation time: 10 minutes Cooking time: 0 minutes

Servings: 4

Ingredients:

1 avocados, pitted, peeled and cut in halves 4 cups vegetable stock

2 tablespoons cilantro, chopped

Juice of 1 lime

1 teaspoon rosemary, dried

½ cup spinach leaves

½ cup kale, torn

Salt and black pepper to the tasteDirections:

In a blender, combine the avocados with the stock and the other ingredients, pulse well, divide into bowls and serve for lunch.

Nutrition: calories 300, fat 23, fiber 5, carbs 6, protein 7

31 Curry spinach soup

Preparation: 10 minutesCooking: 0 minutes Servings: 4

Ingredients:

1 cup almond milk

1 tablespoon green curry paste1 pound spinach leaves

1 tablespoon cilantro, chopped

Salt and black pepper to the taste4 cups veggie stock

1 tablespoon cilantro, choppedDirections:

In your blender, combine the almond milk with the curry paste and the other ingredients, pulse well, divide into bowls and serve for lunch. Nutrition: calories 240, fat 4, fiber 2, carbs 6, protein 2

32 Hot roasted peppers cream

Preparation: 10 minutes Cooking: 30 minutesServings: 4

Ingredients:

1 red chili pepper, minced4 garlic cloves, minced

2 pounds mixed bell peppers, roasted, peeled and

chopped 4 scallions, chopped1 cup coconut cream

Salt and black pepper to the taste2 tablespoons olive oil

½ tablespoon basil, chopped4 cups vegetable stock

¼ cup chives, chopped

Directions:

Heat up a pot with the oil over medium heat, add the

garlic and thechili pepper and sauté for 5 minutes.

Add the peppers and the other ingredients, toss, bring to a simmerand cook over medium heat for 25 minutes.

Blend the soup using an immersion blender, divide into bowls andserve.

Nutrition: calories 140, fat 2, fiber 2, carbs 5, protein 8

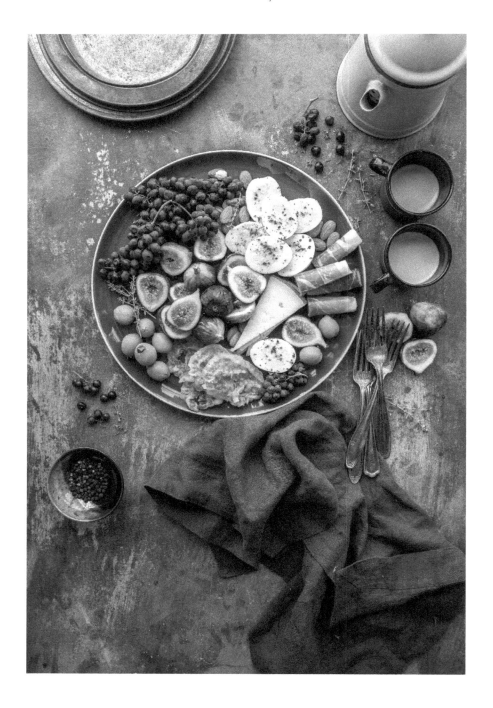

Recipes For Main Courses

And Single Dishes

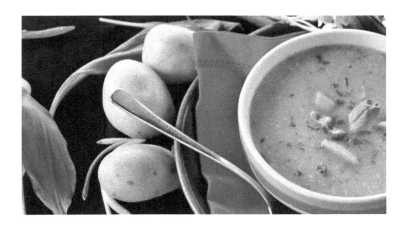

33 Smoked Tempeh with Broccoli Fritters

Preparation Time: 25 minutes Cooking Time: 20 minutes

Servings: 4

Ingredients:

For the flax egg:

4 tbsp flax seed powder + 12 tbsp water For the grilled

tempeh:

3 tbsp olive oil

1 tbsp soy sauce

3 tbsp fresh lime juice1 tbsp grated ginger

Salt and cayenne pepper to taste10 oz. tempeh slices

For the broccoli fritters:

2 cups of rice broccoli8 oz. tofu cheese

3 tbsp plain flour

½ tsp onion powder1 tsp salt

¼ tsp freshly ground black pepper4¼ oz. vegan butter

For serving:

½ cup mixed salad greens1 cup vegan mayonnaise

½ lemon, juicedDirections:

For the smoked tempeh:

In a bowl, mix the flax seed powder with water and set aside to soak for 5 minutes.In another bowl, combine the olive oil, soy sauce, lime juice, grated ginger, salt, and cayenne pepper. Brush the tempeh slices with the mixture.

Heat a grill pan over medium heat and grill the tempeh on both sides until nicely smoked and golden brown, 8 minutes. Transfer to a plate and set aside in a warmer for serving.

In a medium bowl, combine the broccoli rice, tofu cheese,

flour, onion, salt, and black pepper. Mix in the flax egg until well combine and form 1-inch thick patties out of the mixture.

Melt the vegan butter in a medium skillet over medium heat and fry the patties on both sides until golden brown, 8 minutes. Remove the fritters onto a plate and set aside.

In a small bowl, mix the vegan mayonnaise with the lemon juice.

Divide the smoked tempeh and broccoli fritters onto serving plates, add the salad greens, and serve with the vegan mayonnaise sauce.

34 **Cheesy Potato Casserole**

Preparation Time: 30 minutes Cooking Time: 20 minutes

Servings: 4

Ingredients:

2 oz. vegan butter

½ cup celery stalks, finely chopped 1 white onion, finely

chopped

1 green bell pepper, seeded and finely chopped Salt and

black pepper to taste

2 cups peeled and chopped potatoes 1 cup vegan

mayonnaise

4 oz. freshly shredded vegan Parmesan cheese 1 tsp red

chili flakes

Directions:

Preheat the oven to 400 F and grease a baking dish with cookingspray.

Season the celery, onion, and bell pepper with salt and blackpepper.

In a bowl, mix the potatoes, vegan mayonnaise, Parmesan cheese,and red chili flakes.

Pour the mixture into the baking dish, add the season vegetables,and mix well.

Bake in the oven until golden brown, about 20 minutes. Remove the baked potato and serve warm with baby spinach.

35 Curry Mushroom Pie

Preparation Time: 65 minutes Cooking Time: 1 hour

Servings: 4

Ingredients:

For the piecrust:

1 tbsp flax seed powder + 3 tbsp water

¾ cup plain flour 4 tbsp. chia seeds

4 tbsp almond flour

1 tbsp nutritional yeast1 tsp baking powder

1 pinch salt

3 tbsp olive oil4 tbsp water For the filling:

1 cup chopped baby Bella mushrooms 1 cup vegan

mayonnaise

3 tbsp + 9 tbsp water

½ red bell pepper, finely chopped1 tsp curry powder

½ tsp paprika powder ½ tsp garlic powder

¼ tsp black pepper ½ cup coconut cream

1¼ cups shredded vegan Parmesan cheeseDirections:

In two separate bowls, mix the different portions of flaxseed powder with the respective quantity of water. Allow soaking for 5 minutes.

For the piecrust:

Preheat the oven to 350 F.

When the flax egg is ready, pour the smaller quantity into

a food processor and pour in all the ingredients for the piecrust. Blend until soft, smooth dough forms.

Line an 8-inch springform pan with parchment paper and grease withcooking spray.

Spread the dough in the bottom of the pan and bake for 15 minutes.For the filling:

In a bowl, add the remaining flax egg and all the filling's ingredients.Combine well and pour the mixture on the piecrust. Bake further for 40 minutes or until the pie is golden brown.

Remove from the oven and allow cooling for 1 minute.

Slice and serve the pie warm.

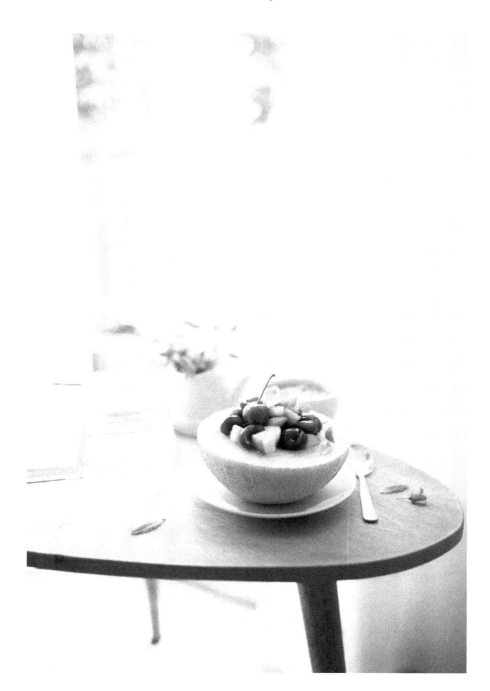

Nutrient-Packed Protein

Salads

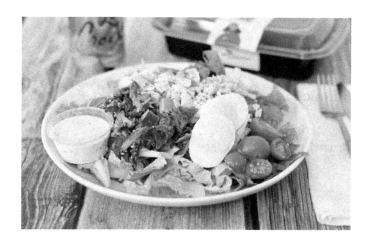

36 Arugula Lentil Salad

Preparation time: 5 mins.Cooking time: 5 mins.

Ingredient: ¾ cups cashews (¾ cups = 100 g)1 onion

3 tbsp olive oil

1 chilli / jalapeño

5-6 sun-dried tomatoes in oil 3 slices bread (whole wheat)

1 cup brown lentils, cooked (1 cup = 1 / 15oz / 400 g)

1 handful arugula/rocket (1 handful = 100 g) 1-2 tbsp balsamic vinegar

salt and pepper to taste.

Directions:

Roast the cashews on a low heat for about three minutes in a pan to maximize aroma. Then throw them into the salad bowl. Dice up and fry the onion in one third of the olive oil for about 3 minutes on a low heat. Meanwhile chop the chilli/jalapeño and dried tomatoes. Add them to the pan and fry for another 1-2 minutes. Cut the bread into big croutons. Move the onion mix into a big bowl. Now add the rest of the oil to the pan and fry the chopped-up bread until crunchy. Season with salt and pepper. Wash the arugula and add it to the bowl. Put the lentils in too, and mix them all around. Season with salt, pepper and balsamic vinegar. Serve with the croutons. Super tasty!

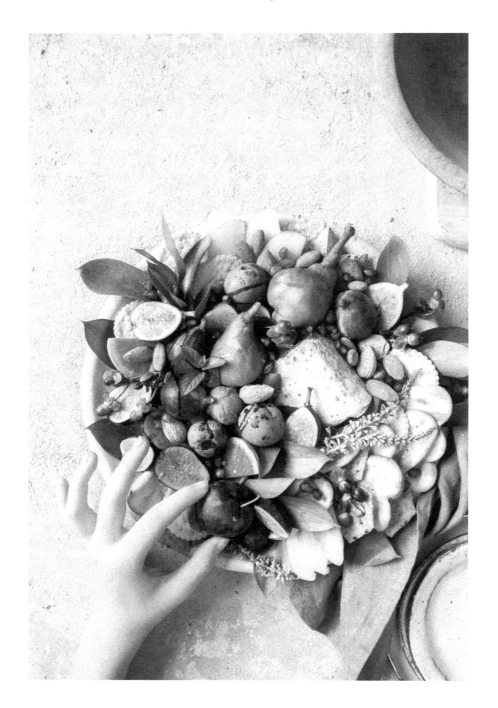

Flavour Boosters (Fish

Glazes, Meat Rubs & Fish

Rubs)

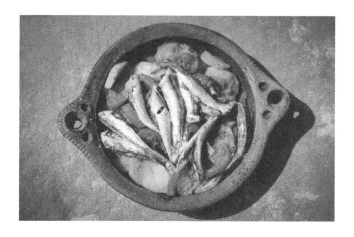

37 Tunisian Mixed Spiced Rub

This incredible rub recipe hailed from the Tunisian

cooking secrets; the rub is the essential seasoning base for variety of Tunisian dishes.

This lovely spice blend created by caraway seeds, coriander, and hot pepper works like a charm on your favorite pork tenderloin, chicken as well as salmon.

Preparation Time: 5 min.Cooking Time: 5 min.

Servings: 5-½ tsp.Ingredients:

Coriander seeds - 2 tsp. Caraway seeds - 2 tsp. Crushed red pepper - 3/4 tsp.Garlic powder - 3/4 tsp.

Kosher salt - 1/2 tsp.Directions:

Mix in the coriander seeds, red pepper and caraway seeds in your spice blender, grinder or processor to make this rub. Start processing or blending the mixed spices on "pulse" mode mixture to ground.

Put the mixed spice mixture into a bowl; mix in the salt and garlic powder. Mix again well.

Now, take your choice of meat cut and place it on a firm surface. Brush or rub the freshly made rub on it; pat gently for the rub to stick onto the surface. Turn the meat cut and repeat to spice up its other side. Repeat with other meat cuts.

The freshly rubbed meat is ready to be grilled or cooked!

38 All Purpose Dill Seed Rub

Boost your steak with vibrant, spiced flavors of this all-purpose dill seed rub. It also beautifully seasons chicken and pork meat cuts. Apply this unique rub minutes before grilling or cooking; you can also store it at room temperature for 12-14 days without sacrificing on its quality.

Preparation Time: 5 min.Cooking Time: 5 min.

Servings: 6-7 tsp.

Ingredients:

Paprika - 2 tsp.

Ground coriander - 2 tsp.Dill seed – 1 tsp.

Dry mustard - ½ tsp. Garlic, minced – 1 clove

Black pepper and salt as requiredCayenne pepper - ¼ tsp.

Directions:

Mix in all the rub ingredients in your mixing bowl to make the dillseed rub. Gently mix all ingredients using spatula or spoon to forman aromatic rub mixture.

Now, take your choice of meat cut and place it on a firm surface. Brush the freshly made rub on it; pat gently for the rub to stick onto the surface. Turn the meat cut and repeat to spice up its other side. Repeat with other meat cuts.

Let your meat cuts adequately season for more rich flavors for a few hours in your refrigerator. Take them out, as they are ready to be cooked or grilled!

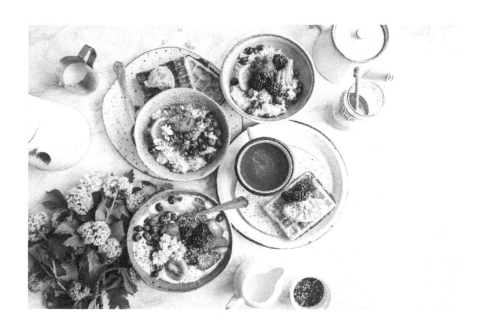

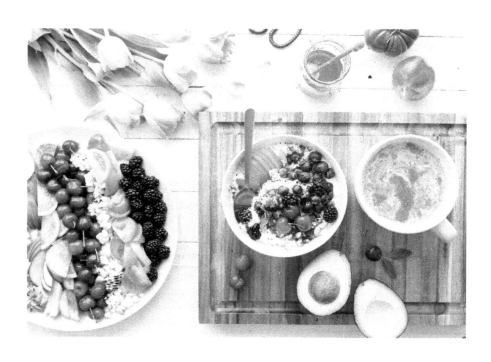

Sauce Recipes

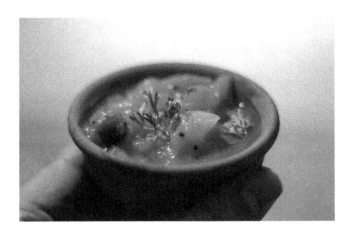

39 Vegan Ranch Dressing (Dipping Sauce)

Preparation time: 5 minutes Cooking time: 5 minutes

Servings: 8

Ingredients:

1 tablespoons lemon juice14 oz. silken tofu

1 tablespoon yellow mustard

1 tablespoon apple cider vinegar1 teaspoon onion granules

1 tablespoon agave

1 teaspoon garlic granules

2 tablespoons parsley, minced2 tablespoons dill, minced

1/2 teaspoon Himalayan salt

Directions:

Add all ingredients except parsley and dill to a blender and blenduntil smooth at high speed.

Add dill and parsley and blend until mixed.Serve chilled.

40 Vegan Smokey Maple BBQ Sauce

Preparation time: 5 minutes Cooking time: 5 minutes

Servings: 8

Ingredients:

1 tablespoon maple syrup1/2 cup ketchup

1 teaspoon garlic powder 1 teaspoon liquid smoke

Directions:

Add all ingredients to a bowl. Mix them until well combined.Serve and enjoy.

CPSIA information can be obtained
at www.ICGtesting.com
Printed in the USA
LVHW081314150521
687183LV00045B/755

9 781802 890662